Health Systems Engineering: Building A Better Healthcare Delivery System

Mbuso Mabuza

Published by Lekwandza Media, 2023.

While every precaution has been taken in the preparation of this book, the publisher assumes no responsibility for errors or omissions, or for damages resulting from the use of the information contained herein.

HEALTH SYSTEMS ENGINEERING: BUILDING A BETTER HEALTHCARE DELIVERY SYSTEM

First edition. May 27, 2023.

ISBN: 979-8223879367

Written by Mbuso Mabuza.

Also by Mbuso Mabuza

A Healthy Mind And Best You: Achieving Great Results in Every Aspect of Your Life
Purposeful And Better You
Sustainable Development Calls for Effective Strategic Leadership for Efficient Health Systems
Health Promotion In Low Socioeconomic Settings
Medicine and Sociology of Health
Qualitative Methods In Public Health Research
Global Health Disaster Management
Global Health Policy And Programme Challenges
The Journey of Life Has a Gift of Purpose
Epidemiological Research
Ethics, Qualitative And Quantitative Methods In Public Health Research
When Love Lasts
Blockchain Technology In Healthcare
Virtual and Augmented Reality in Healthcare
Data Analytics and Healthcare Informatics
How To Improve The Way You Think
Health Systems Engineering: Building A Better Healthcare Delivery System
Artificial Intelligence In Drug Discovery And Development

Table of Contents

Preface

There is increasing recognition that efforts to improve global health cannot be achieved without stronger health systems.

The myriad of opportunities and challenges that come with rapid technological innovations in the medical and health ecosystem, warrant an urgent need to apply systems engineering techniques and skills to solve issues pertaining to healthcare service quality, patient safety, and healthcare cost, as means to improve healthcare systems performance. Health systems engineering can solve healthcare problems that no one else can.

Health systems engineering entails the application of engineering, science, management, and technological innovation to healthcare systems improvement. A successful systems engineering delivery process in healthcare should focus on defining stakeholder needs and required functionality early in the development cycle, documenting requirements, then proceeding with design synthesis and system validation while considering the complete problem. It focuses on understanding the interactions among people (patients, families, clinicians, and other stakeholders), processes (institutional, regulatory, professional ethics, etc.), and technology (medical devices and instrumentation) in the healthcare domain to formulate a systems approach to innovations that lead to improved patient outcomes.

The needs of the patient and family are not limited to improved communication but also extend beyond what people commonly consider technology-related topics. The proposed healthcare setting should have the environmental factors desired by patients and family members as expressed by them, suggesting a need for improvements in the healthcare environment. The patient and family must be kept at the centre of the systems approach. There are no technical barriers to enabling that capability, and the payoff in terms of patient and family experience may be substantial.

Perhaps, health is too important to be left only to doctors; the healthcare consumer's well-being should be the primary consideration. The ultimate goal is to ensure that quality goals and objectives of the 21st century health system are achieved through accessible, safe, effective, patient-centred, timely, efficient, and equitable health care.

There is no doubt that very few healthcare professionals or administrators are equipped to think analytically about health care delivery as a system or to appreciate the relevance of systems engineering tool. Even fewer are equipped to work to apply these tools. With the increasing global burden of disease, and the risk of pandemics such as we have already seen with the COVID-19, there is an urgent need to develop and enhance capacity for the design and application of health systems engineering, in order to build a better healthcare delivery system. A very important issue therefore is for the educators, students and practitioners to develop a sound understanding of what health systems engineering actually means. Accordingly, there is a need for multi-skilled professionals with qualifications in health systems engineering.

This book aims to address that need. The book begins with an overview of a systems approach to healthcare. It then discusses health systems including health systems strengthening and the role of knowledge management and leadership, essential health packages, public-private partnerships, healthcare financing, and monitoring performance. Health systems engineering is discussed with a particular focus on engineering better health and care, and on how it can transform the medical and healthcare ecosystem. This book will appeal to professionals and students in medicine and healthcare, global health, public health, health economics, healthcare leadership and management, health systems strengthening and research, healthcare innovations, data analytics and health informatics, systems engineering, sustainable development, public policy, social sciences, and related fields.

Chapter 1

A Systems Approach to Healthcare

"Systems that work do not just happen – they have to be planned, designed and built." – Coulter, 2005

———◦———

OVER THE PAST TWO TO three decades, there have been numerous calls to implement a more holistic systems approach to transform health and care to address the needs of a changing patient population. However, there has been no clear definition of what this might mean in practice.

A systems approach maintains a perspective in which the overall effectiveness and efficiency in achieving objectives depends on identification, understanding, and management of interrelated processes as a collective system. This description of a systems approach raises the question: what is a system? The International Council of Systems Engineering (INCOSE) offers this sound definition of a system:

A system is a construct or collection of different elements that together produce results not obtainable by the elements alone. The elements, or parts, can include people, hardware, software, facilities, policies, and documents; that is, all things required to produce systems-level results. The results include system level qualities, properties, characteristics, functions, behaviour and performance. The value added by the system as a whole, beyond that contributed independently by the parts, is primarily created by the relationship among the parts; that is, how they are interconnected.

Armed with this definition of a system, we can expand on the systems approach concept by requiring the following:

- Definition of the objectives or goals of the system
- Elaboration of the interdependencies between the processes of the system
- Clarification of the roles of the constituent system elements necessary to achieve objectives (thereby reducing cross-functional barriers)
- Definition of the system's capabilities
- Establishment of performance expectations prior to operational employment
- Measurement and evaluation of performance to continually improve the system through measurement and evaluation.

Using a systems approach as a lens to look at today's health care "system" makes it readily apparent that health care as it exists today is neither a system nor a system of systems. Healthcare as a whole is not managed as a set of interrelated processes. The interdependencies among the constituent elements (everything from devices to electronic medical records, from in-patient care to home care, etc.) are loosely defined at best. Cross-sectional boundaries abound in health care settings – the boundaries exist between patients and the clinical team, within the clinical team itself, between the patient and the patient's family, and between the operators of medical devices and the devices themselves. The current model of medical delivery generates an abundance of data, but the system often fails to generate actionable information. This failure to produce information results in an inability to establish meaningful performance expectations or to permit measurement and evaluation (Johns Hopkins University, 2013).

Engineers routinely use a systems approach to address challenging problems in complex projects. This allows them to work through the implications of each change or decision they make for the project as a whole. They consider the layout of the system, defining all the elements and interconnections, to ensure that the whole system performs as required.

All health and care improvement initiatives involve people, processes, technologies, the physical environment and systems that, in turn, are part of other systems. For example, the care pathway of an elderly frail patient must meet the needs of the patient, their immediate carer and wider family. Care must also coordinate across community support, a physician's practice and hospital teams, and manage the patient's medication, their physical journey to and around healthcare facilities, home care technologies and associated health and care data. Such complexity means that health and care will benefit from using an approach that considers each relevant element of the system and, critically, the nature and performance of the interfaces between them.

There is potential for health and care improvement to benefit from the rigour of the engineering approach to systems, particularly with respect to: systems being centred on people; iteration before implementation; design as an exploratory process; and risk management as a proactive process.

While pockets of excellence exist in the use of a systems approach in healthcare, the common sense thinking presented here is still far from being common practice.

A systems approach can be defined and applied in a health and care context as a series of questions that integrate people, systems, design, and risk perspectives in an ordered and well executed manner. It is only when all four are robustly understood and considered that a systems approach will have the greatest success.

All improvement initiatives involve people, processes, technologies and systems that, in turn, are part of other systems. This complexity means that all parts of the health and care system stand to benefit from using an approach which considers each relevant element of the overall system and joins them up efficiently.

A true systems approach is one that consistently delivers a high-quality service and is most likely to be the result of a team successfully integrating people, systems, design, and risk perspectives in an ordered and well executed manner.

A system (or system of systems) is a set of elements: people, processes, information, organisations and services, as well as software, hardware and other systems that, when combined, have qualities that are not present in any of the elements themselves.

A system is delineated by its spatial and temporal boundaries, surrounded and influenced by its environment, described by its structure and purpose, and expressed in its functioning. In other words, the whole is very likely to be greater than the sum of the parts.

A systems approach uses a range of techniques to determine requirements for the system, organise its structure, create and evaluate alternative designs, produce quantitative analyses and predictions where appropriate, assess possible threats to and opportunities for people and other systems, integrate all the individual elements and delivery system that is shown to be fit for its intended purpose. A true systems approach does not deliver solely technical solutions; rather it ensures the appropriate alignment of technology, processes, interactions and policy to deliver innovative responses to today's most complex and pressing challenges.

A systems approach can be applied to the design and improvement of systems across many areas of health and care.

A systems approach can be applied to the design and improvement of systems at all extremes of scale, with service level improvement taking place within a wider context that may subsequently require changes at the organisation level and cross-organisational level. Within the delivery of health and care, many systems are distinct and can be operated independently, yet are also connected to or integrated with other systems, either in layers or as part of a network. The strength of a systems approach is its ability to overcome the complexity associated with such systems of systems and deliver solutions at all levels of scale regardless of the form of the system. Its value has been recognised in health and care and increasingly referred to in national policies and used in improvement methods.

A systems approach aims to determine the system design and implementation that delivers the best service. It has the potential to drive greater efficiency and a better understanding of threats and opportunities present when shaping the delivery of health and care services. A systems approach brings together four key and complementary perspectives:

People: understanding of interactions among people, at the personal, group and organisational levels, and other elements of a system in order to improve overall system performance (identify, locate, situate).

- Who will use the system (identify)?
- Where is the system (locate)?
- What affects the system (situate)?

Systems: addressing complex and uncertain real world problems, involving highly interconnected technical and social elements that typically produce emergent properties and behaviour (understand, organise, and integrate).

- Who are the stakeholders (understand)?
- What are the elements (organise)?
- How does the system perform (integrate)?

Design: focusing on improvement by identifying the right problem to solve, creating a range of possible solutions and refining the best of these to deliver appropriate outcomes (explore, create, evaluate).

- What are the needs (explore)?
- How can the needs be met (create)?

- How well are the needs met (evaluate)?

Risk: managing risk, based on the timely identification of threats and opportunities in the system, assessment of their associated risks and management of necessary change (examine, assess, and improve).

- What is going on (examine)?
- What could go wrong (assess)?
- How can we make it better (improve)?

All these perspectives are inextricably linked and uniquely contribute to a systems approach. It is only when all four are robustly understood that a systems approach will have the greatest success.

Improvement initiatives involve people and systems that, in turn, are inevitably part of other systems. Consequently, they would all stand to benefit from using a systems approach that delivers coordinated improvement to all the systems.

All improvement initiatives should start with the question:

Why are we doing this? – leads to a documented rationale for improving an existing system or developing a new one (trigger).

The trigger defines the entry point for any subsequent improvement process and may be the result of:

- **Strategic development:** where risk reduction and improvement is part of an ongoing strategic initiative.
- **An incident:** where an event has resulted in actual or potential harm to patients or clinicians
- **Local concerns:** where the potential for incidents has been identified through general observation or evidenced by data trends
- **Routine service review:** where a team or individual wishes to check the integrity of their service
- **Service improvement:** where national, regional or local

changes are planned to an existing service or system

- **New service:** where a new service is to be introduced into practice or an existing one decommissioned
- **Technology introduction:** where new equipment or technology is to be introduced to an existing service
- **Building or estate changes:** where estates or buildings are being built, refurbished or maintained
- **Staff changes:** where new staff are to be introduced to an existing service or existing staff levels are changed
- **External directive:** where specific strategic changes or checks are requested
- **National initiatives:** where teams are encouraged to propose and deliver service improvements.

A clear understanding of the trigger helps to identify the initial scope of the improvement and ensures that an appropriate team is assembled to initiate any subsequent improvement process. Whether the trigger relates to people, systems, design or risk, a systems approach will consider all of these perspectives in a seamless and integrated way. This leads onto a final ongoing challenge:

What should we do next? – leads to the ongoing development and execution of a plan of action to deliver the system in a timely manner (plan).

Systems thinking for health systems strengthening offers a practical approach to improving health systems through a systems thinking lens. It works to reveal the underlying characteristics and relationships of systems which are described as dynamic architectures of interactions and synergies. Such systems typically exhibit non-linear and unpredictable behaviour, are resistant to change, and provide a challenge where seemingly obvious solutions can worsen a problem.

The systems thinking framework describes ten practical steps in a two-stage conceptual process that can be adapted to many different situations. Intervention design includes convening stakeholders, brainstorming, predicting performance, and adaptation and redesign. Evaluation design includes identification of indicators, choice of methods, selection of design, planning, budgeting and funding.

The Change Model is an organising framework for sustainable change and transformation that delivers potential benefits for patients and the public. As a way of thinking, the model is relevant to numerous change programmes and provides an approach that can be tailored to fit individual situations. It is a way of making sense at every level of the 'how and why' of delivering improvement, to consistently make a bigger difference.

The model has eight components that lead to a better understanding of how to create an environment and programme(s) that can make change happen:

- Our shared purpose
- Leadership by all
- Spread and adoption
- Improvement tools
- Project and performance management
- Measurement
- Influencing factors
- Motivate and mobilise

References

Coulter, A. (2015) What do patients and the public want from primary care? *British Medical Journal*, 331(7526), 1199-1201.

Clinical Human Factors Group (2013) Implementing human factors in healthcare, 'taking further steps'. Clinical Human Factors Group.

Dekker, S.W.A. & Leveson, N.G. (2015) The systems approach to medicine: controversy and misconceptions, *British Medical Journal*, 247, 7-9.

Erwin, K. & Krishnana, J.A.A (2016) Redesigning healthcare to fit with people. *British Medical Journal*, 354(i4536).

Hollnage, I.E., Wears, R. & Braithwaite, J. (2015) From safety-I to Safetyy-II: A White Ppaer. The Resilient Health Care Net: Published simultaneously by the University of Southern Denmark, University of Florida, USA, and Macquarie University, Australia.

Kurtz, C.F. & Snowden, D.J. (2003) The new dynamics of strategy sense-making in a complex world. *IBM Systems Journal*, 42(3), 462-483.

MxGuire, K.J. & Spears, S.J. (2015) Beyond the jargon: architecture, process and clinical care, *SPINE*, 40(16), 1243-1246.

NHS England (2015) New care models: empowering patients and communities, a call to action for a directory of support. NHS England, Redditch, UK.

RAEng (2007) Creating systems that work: principles of engineering systems for the 21st century. Royal Academy of Engineering, London, UK.

Ravitz, A.D., et al. (2013) Systems approach and systems engineering applied to health care: improving patient safety and health care delivery. *Johns Hopkins APL Technical Digest*, 21(4).

The Health Foundation (2013) Quality improvement made simple: what everyone should know about health care quality improvement. The Health Foundation, London.

Chapter 2
Health Systems

*"The sheer size and complexity of a health system, as well as the pressures it faces from an increasing burden of disease and finite resources, mean that making improvements to health and care can be a significant challenge. Successful transformation must take into account the needs of all patients, carers, healthcare professionals and other staff. It requires consistent consideration of every element of the system, the way each element interact, and the implications of these interactions for the system as a whole – that is, it requires a 'systems' approach." – **Rt Hon Professor Lord Darzi of Denham, 2017**

2.1 Introduction

HEALTH SYSTEMS ENCOMPASS all the entities and means whose primary goal is to improve the health of individuals and the population (World Health Organization, 2000). Crucially, health systems carry out service provision, resource generation, financing and stewardship, with the overall goals of achieving good health, responsiveness to the expectations of the population, and fairness of financial contribution (World Health Organization, 2000).

There is increasing recognition that efforts to improve global health cannot be achieved without stronger health systems. Interpretation of health systems strengthening has varied widely however, with much of the focus to-date on alleviating input constraints, whereas less attention has been given to other performance drivers. Many funders of global health initiatives supporting the health system focus on ensuring necessary inputs for the effective delivery of a single or limited set of interventions – vertical programmes. This approach has been accused of creating silos and fragmenting the health system.

The World Health Organization framework, in contrast, looks across interventions and organises the health system into six building blocks or functions, namely: leadership and governance, health financing; service delivery; health workforce; health information; medical technologies (including medical products, vaccines, and other technologies) (World Health Organization, 2007; World Health Organization, 2000). Although this approach cuts across the vertical disease programmes, it too can fragment the health system, albeit by function rather than by disease. The building blocks also further tendencies to segment and limit interventions, under-recognising the complex and cross-cutting nature of health system constraints.

There is increasing recognition of the trade-off between applying immediate solutions that do not strengthen the existing infrastructure/system and making investments that may take longer to reap health benefits, but are more likely to have a lasting impact. Both approaches are important, and must be balanced appropriately, to achieve global health and development goals. As such, strengthening the health system is accomplished by more comprehensive changes to performance drivers such as policies and regulations, organisational structures, and relationships across the health system to motivate changes in behaviour and/or allow more effective use of resources to improve multiple health services (Chee et al, 2013).

The increasing burden of disease and the emergence and re-emergence of infectious diseases, could be catastrophic if not addressed as a matter of urgency. Are health systems in a position to deal with the increasing burden of disease and the emerging pandemics such as COVID-19?

The recent COVID-19 pandemic is testimony to the frailties of health systems, both from a local and global perspective. The magnitude of the global epidemic of non-communicable diseases such as diabetes mellitus, cardiovascular diseases, chronic respiratory diseases, and cancer, continues to rise especially in low- and middle-income countries, and this poses a huge threat on health systems.

———⊖———

2.2 Health systems strengthening and the role of knowledge management and leadership

THE WHO (2000) ACKNOWLEDGES that leadership or stewardship is ultimately concerned with the oversight of the entire health system, and that healthcare financing is the main challenge facing low- and middle-income countries. It can be deduced that the main channels through which the health system is affected are through leadership and its impact on healthcare financing and related effects such as multi-stakeholder harmonisation and service delivery.

Fragmented and poorly led health systems are a silent killer as they cause more sickness and disproportionate numbers of deaths within populations just as in epidemics (Dwyer and Wilhelmsen, n.d.).

Although it is often technically and medically known what is required to reduce illness and to save lives, but what is often lacking is the dearth of knowledge and skills to lead and manage the complexities of health systems (Dwyer and Wilhelmsen, n.d.).

Evidence shows that there is lack of an enabling environment for health systems leadership to flourish, particularly in the low- and middle-income countries such as in sub-Saharan Africa, and this calls for a disruption in the status quo (Gilson and Agyepong, 2018).

Typically, current leadership practices are a barrier to health systems strengthening as they tend to show features of authoritarian rather than participatory leadership style, decision-making is largely centralised or individualised, and the dominance of medical professionals is an impediment to progress (Gilson and Agyepong, 2018). Such a status quo is a recipe for disaster because it could exacerbate the fragility of the other key building blocks of health systems.

"Knowledge management (has potential for maximising results through continuous assessment, capture, synthesis, generation, and sharing of relevant information and knowledge) – connecting the right people to the right data, information, and knowledge at the right time – is increasingly being considered as an effective approach to help strengthen health systems" (USAID, 2012). For example, in the finance building block of the health system, knowledge management ensures that a health system has adequate funds, and can potentially help identify barriers to service access.

As such, the management of this knowledge will affect individual lives, whole communities, and, ultimately, the health, social, and economic status of the entire world. "Studies show that global health organisations that adopt knowledge management strategies and practices can strengthen the performance of health care workers and programmes, and, therefore, leveraging the power of knowledge management can transform global health and development" (Sullivan et al, 2015).

Leadership literature identifies leadership as a central pillar for health systems strengthening, in terms of improving the priority areas of access, quality and utilisation, to ensure sustainability and positive impact (Alva, Kleinau, Pomeroy and Rowan, 2009; Opio et al, 2010). As such, there has been a growing realisation that all leaders in healthcare should have the skills and competency to lead. This includes the ability to scan for opportunities and resources, focus on priority areas, alignment and mobilisation, inspiring, planning, organising, implementing, monitoring and evaluation.

Effective leadership is the sine qua non for achieving maximum impact from health investments at global, national and local levels, yet, this vital pillar is often missing (Quick, 2011). Much as it is laudable that the World Health Organization (WHO) recently issued a statement calling all countries to make three specific commitments to universal health coverage, and be prepared to announce them at the World Health Assembly scheduled for 21 May 2018, such commitments are not enough, unless health systems are strengthened (Eghan, 2018).

An eight-year retrospective study aimed at evaluating the leadership training program within the Centres for Disease Control and Prevention, revealed that such a program had a positive impact on the participants' leadership effectiveness (Woltring et al, 2003). However, it can be argued that such leadership effectiveness was more about how the participants felt after the training process rather than the impact of their leadership, in practice. It can also be argued that with the rapidly changing healthcare environment, leadership skills and competencies, alone, do not guarantee better health outcomes (Jooste, 2009).

In that regard, the WHO (2007) suggested a framework that included leadership competencies, adequate numbers of trained leaders, an enabling working environment, and functional support systems. The good thing about having such a framework is that it provides a structure of what needs to be done so that there could be accountability of leadership's implementation of policy.

However, the WHO framework for leadership and management strengthening in health systems appears to overlook the contextual factors such as how to deal with unique complexities of each specific environment. The application of such a framework and the impact of leadership in specific settings could be a challenge. In most instances, leaders know what to do, in theory, but the application or implementation is always a challenge.

The leadership theories, models or frameworks have been criticised because they are generic instead of being context-specific, bearing in mind that regions, countries and districts are unique, and one glove does not fit all. Theories, models or frameworks are useful as a point of reference, but they should not be prescriptive and static, they should be relevant and evolving, in line with the constantly changing healthcare landscape.

Heading (2009) puts it succinctly in a discussion paper which highlights that the changing health systems environment requires more than a mechanistic approach, but a consideration of broader influences and local issues. As such, leadership strengthening of health systems should consider a mix of leadership traits, behaviours, tools, and contextual factors (Heading, 2009).

Global Health Leadership

The Report of the G8 Health Experts Group (2009) acknowledges the global health leadership mandate that the WHO has, as well as the financial global health dominance of the World Bank. The strength of the report is that it highlights the need to reposition and strengthen global health leadership, in line with the changing landscape of global health architecture, bearing in mind the limitations of WHO and the World Bank (The Report of the G8 Health Experts Group, 2009).

The WHO, operating within the United Nations, responsible for global health leadership and governance, produced a report with comparisons and rankings of different health systems (Smith and Papanicolas, 2004). The comparison and ranking of health systems serves the purpose of benchmarking so that strengths and weaknesses could be highlighted from which lessons could be learnt for better performance (Kumar and Ozdamar, 2004). However, the weaknesses of such comparisons were the methodological challenges that were inherent in such comparisons as health systems differ from a contextual and cultural perspective (Kelley, Arispe and Holmes, 2006). There was also the dilemma of how the findings should be communicated to the policymakers, and how such findings should be used by the policymakers of the different countries (Kelley, Arispe and Holmes, 2006).

The World Health Report 2000 acknowledges that leadership or stewardship is ultimately concerned with the oversight of the entire health system, and that healthcare financing is the main challenge facing low- and middle-income countries (Dare and Reeler, 2005; WHO, 2000). The World Health Report placed leadership on the lap of national authorities or policy makers to ensure that policies are implemented and that there are specific indicators for better performance of health systems (WHO, 2000). It also placed the responsibility on leadership to ensure that there is effective healthcare financing to enable equitable healthcare access by all (WHO, 2000). However, the WHO report was oblivious of the uniqueness of each country and the complexity of the roles that multiple stakeholders such as the private sector, NGOs, and development or donor agencies could play in the health system.

In an assessment of the World Health Report 2000, Navarro (2000) argued against the report's mechanistic view of health systems strengthening. Such mechanistic view focused on the "conventional wisdom" of "magic bullets" to fix the health systems challenges from a government's perspective, and overlooked the social, economic, and political dynamics of each country (Navarro, 2000). There is need to have a better understanding of leadership's successes and challenges in the health sector so that context-specific solutions could be developed, bearing in mind the multiple stakeholders in the context of each setting.

A summary of the debate at the Special Session on Future Directions in Health Care Financing held at the 6th Congress of the International Health Economics Association (iHEA) highlighted the knowledge gap pertaining to healthcare financing in low- and middle-income countries (Danish Ministry of Foreign Affairs, 2007). Such a debate was an eye opener because the main focus was on major funding mechanisms that could sustain healthcare financing in the context of both developed and developing countries. However, the weakness of the debate was that it was based on existing studies which were conducted in developed countries because of the paucity of studies conducted in developing countries (Ataguba and Akazili, 2010). It would be interesting to explore how leadership's increased focus on specific disease programmes such as

HIV and AIDS, tuberculosis, and malaria has affected the opportunity cost of addressing other urgent health matters such as the escalating epidemic of non-communicable diseases, and the need for investing in innovation and technology in changing the future of healthcare in disease high burden countries and regions.

A retrospective and prospective analysis of the 2014 West African Ebola epidemic highlights lack of budget as a limitation of WHO (Gostin and Friedman, 2014). Lack of legal framework to interact with the public sector, private sector, NGOs and development agencies is highlighted as another weakness of WHO (Gostin and Friedman, 2014; The Report of the G8 Health Experts Group, 2009).

According to an article by Montegut (2007), the other limitation of WHO has been the disease-focused vertical approach to global healthcare instead of a broad-based horizontal approach. Other authors argue that a combination of vertical and horizontal approaches and flexibility to suite each particular context could be the best approach (The Report of the G8 Health Experts Group, 2009).

The fundamental structural changes of the global health architecture of the 21st century have been characterised by the emergence of influential stakeholders in the global health leadership arena. Stakeholders such as the Bill & Melinda Gates Foundation, GAVI, and the Global Fund, have come at the back of a declining prior dominance of WHO and the World Bank (The Report of the G8 Health Experts Group, 2009).

The embracing of global health by the G8, and the emergence of the Health 8 or H8 provides a locus for discussion on global health policy and an opportunity for collaborative global health leadership efforts. However, the weakness is that the G8 has lack of capacity, and the H8 is still trying to find its role in the global health leadership milieu (The Report of the G8 Health Experts Group, 2009). It can be argued that since the G8 comprises leaders of the advanced market economies, how could the health agenda for middle- and low-income countries be decided by a few rich countries? Perhaps, this point of view calls for purposefulness, organisation and synergy between an empowered and more effective WHO at the top and sustainable, equitable national health systems at the root core (Gostin and Friedman, 2014).

There is an increasing need to define, understand and manage the global health system amidst the challenges of globalisation (Johnson and Stoskopf, 2010). The constantly changing global health landscape requires leaders to have joint commitment and eyes to see and act on global health challenges that are happening now, and eyes to see and act on global health challenges that will happen in the future (Fried et al, 2012). It requires global health leaders to walk the talk, to have new thinking and new ways of doing and acting to address current global health challenges and to prevent future challenges (Fried et al, 2012).

———◉———

2.3 Essential health packages

ESSENTIAL MEDICAL LABORATORY services could provide evidence-based recommendations to support essential health packages (EHPs) (Dacombe et al, 2006). There are different interpretations of EHPs, but in general they could be defined in the context of a sector-wide approach as aspirational or short term tools meant to apportion tailored, cost effective health services, aimed at addressing health priorities, and are sometimes considered as a safety net for the poor or vulnerable populations (Ensor et al, 2002; World Health Organization, 2008).

Implementation of essential medical laboratory services has some constraints such as in Malawi as highlighted below (Dacombe et al, 2006).

Constraints:

- Policymakers' lack of understanding of the resource

requirements of a functional laboratory and how a laboratory functions, and health workers' lack of awareness of vital diagnostic approaches to EHP conditions (Dacombe et al, 2006; Mueller et al, 2011).

- Screening blood for infections can be very costly especially if the "gold standard" methods are employed such as light microscopy for detection of malaria parasites, and sputum-smear microscopy for detection of TB bacilli, as these are difficult to provide in the remote settings as such screenings require huge investments in high level technical expertise, quality monitoring and equipment maintenance which are lacking at the primary care level (Dacombe et al, 2006)
- The magnitude of the problem such as high prevalence of blood-borne infections in in Malawi could overwhelm the capacity of the laboratory services (Dacombe et al, 2006).
- Patients and their relatives may have to travel far to have their blood screened in a district laboratory, and this may be an added burden not only on the sick but on households of the sick as well in terms of transport costs and poor infrastructure (Dacombe et al, 2006)
- The community's negative perception of the laboratory services could result in underutilisation of the laboratory services (Derua et al, 2011).

Possible solutions:

- It would be crucial to assess and collect locally relevant evidence about the needs of the communities and the feasibility of providing laboratory services to address those needs and to support the delivery of an essential health package (Dacombe et al, 2006)
- Effective leadership and human capacity building as well as adequate equipment and supplies could address the issue of the

magnitude of the demand for laboratory testing due to the huge disease burden in certain settings (Ndihokubwayo et al, 2010).

- Improving the quality of care and standards of the laboratory services through internal quality assurance linked to external quality assurance mechanisms could improve efficiency and also address the issue of the public's negative perception of the laboratory services (Dacombe et al, 2006)
- Bringing the laboratory services into the primary care setting could be more feasible and could relieve the burden on laboratories at the secondary level of care, and could also be easily accessible to the community (Dacombe et al, 2006)
- Provision of rapid diagnostic tests such as for anaemia, HIV, antenatal syphilis, and malaria could be more feasible and less costly when provided at the primary care setting (Dacombe et al, 2006).

Effective essential medical laboratory services are crucial as part of an integrated EHP (Dacombe et al, 2006). However, greater attention needs to be given to removing the constraints of delivering effective medical laboratory services to support EHPs (Dacombe et al, 2006).

In a number of sub-Saharan African countries, lack of knowledge, understanding and awareness of laboratory functions by policymakers, health professional and patients is so pronounced that it stifles progress towards delivering cost-effective and equitable health services. There is an urgent need for policymakers, health professionals and patients that are both informed and active (Haines, Kuruvilla and Borchert, 2004).

The starting point should be the strengthening of institutions and mechanisms that can more systematically promote interactions between researchers, policy-makers and other stakeholders who can influence the process (Haines, Kuruvilla and Borchert, 2004). Finding more effective ways of increasing knowledge and understanding about essential medical laboratory services to support health services delivery should be a priority for researchers, health professionals and policy-makers (Haines, Kuruvilla and Borchert, 2004). Even when the evidence and systematic ways of increasing knowledge and understanding are available, further work is needed to translate it into guidelines or messages that are understandable to patients and health professionals (Haines, Kuruvilla and Borchert, 2004).

Training health professionals at institutions of higher learning should be structured in such a way that it equips them with core competencies and skills that will enable them to face the real challenges of implementing essential health packages including essential medical laboratory services (Pruitt and Epping-Jordan, 2005). Promoting interdepartmental collaboration such as in the training curricula of doctors, nurses, and medical laboratory professionals will require increasing the capacity of institutions of higher learning (Mullan et al, 2011). It is encouraging that the innovative educational approach that integrates leadership and management training into the traditional medical curricula in Botswana, could enhance the employability of policymakers and health professionals that are well informed (Magowe et al, 2014).

Mitton et al (2007) suggest the use of new technologies such as knowledge transfer and exchange (KTE) which is an interactive exchange of knowledge between research users and research producers with the primary purpose of increasing the likelihood that research evidence will be used in policy and practice decisions. Drummond et al (2008) add that health technology assessments (HTAs) can be used to inform policymakers by using the best evidence-based information to inform best practices in health care service delivery. Such new technologies could enhance or increase policymakers' knowledge and understanding of essential medical laboratory services.

However, it is worth noting that implementing new technologies could be a challenge in low-income countries, as low-income countries face additional challenges to using research evidence due to weak health systems, lack of professional regulation and lack of access to evidence (Haines, Kuruvilla and Borchert, 2004). Jasser highlights an important point about contextualising interventions and training to the setting (Bheekie, Adonis and Daniels, 2009). More than ever before the world needs comprehensive responses to complex problems (Frenk, 2006).

Interestingly, there have been creative solutions for the implementation of medical laboratory services in low- and middle-income countries such as Uganda. The wide coverage, cost-effectiveness and consistency of the HUB specimen Transport Network System appears to be the answer to addressing the non-sustainable previously implemented specimen transport methods via the post office (Kiyaga et al, 2013).

Since low- and middle-income countries are often acutely challenged when it comes to implementing sustainable health care interventions, the specimen Transport Network System that was successfully implemented in Uganda is a model for efficiency in low- and middle income countries (Go Molecular, n.d.). The success of such an efficient laboratory services revolved around effective leadership, planning, coordination and innovation, among others.

It has been fascinating to see the Greater Sekhukhune-CAPABILITY Outreach Project that was undertaken in a rural district in Limpopo, South Africa, aimed at initiating a district clinical genetic service including a medical laboratory service to gain knowledge and experience to assist in the implementation and development of medical genetic services in South Africa (Gregersen et al, 2013). It is worth noting that this initiative was impeded by a developing staff shortage in the province and pressure on the health service from the existing HIV/AIDS and TB epidemics (Gregersen et al, 2013).

However, these impediments stimulated the pioneering of innovative ways to offer medical genetic services in these circumstances including tele-teaching of nurses and doctors, using cellular phones to enhance clinical care and adapting and assessing the clinical utility of a laboratory test, QF-PCR, for use in the local circumstances (Gregersen et al, 2013).

What this tells me is that sometimes, in the midst of a challenge or constraint there is a solution, and at the same time such a solution should be context-specific in order to ensure that there is cost-effectiveness of the intervention. Constraints during the implementation of health interventions could also be an opportunity to learn and to go back to the drawing board to be able to come up with more feasible approaches to effectively deliver health services.

Although some concerns have been raised about lack of electricity in the rural areas of many low- and middle income countries which makes it difficult to implement new health technologies, such issues can be addressed through adding applications and accessory attachments to mobile phones that turn them into diagnostic tools (Mossman et al, 2014). In the case of "Health Care at My Fingertips" in Kenya, programs are using wireless e-health tablets to take high resolution photographs and perform diagnostic evaluations (Mossman et al, 2014).

Whilst essential health packages (EHPs) have increasingly been considered as an important tool of health policy in terms of cost-effectively addressing health priorities in accordance with the local burden of disease, the mechanisms of delivery of essential health packages have often been overlooked (Mueller et al, 2011).

It is a limitation on its own to overlook the mechanisms of delivery of essential health packages as this could fail to achieve what the essential health packages are intended for, and could also incur unnecessary costs and defeat the very essence of essential health packages which is to deliver rationed health services cost-effectively and equitably (WHO, 2008).

There is need for clear understanding, scope, purpose, level of delivery and the shape of the delivery of the essential health service, otherwise the implementation of the essential health package would be limited or constrained (Victora et al, 2004; WHO, 2008). It is a limitation if the implemented essential health packages end up only benefiting those who can afford, whilst the poor and vulnerable have considerable barriers to accessing such services (Ensor et al, 2002). Shortage of essential medicines is another limitation that could hamper the implementation of the EHPs (Greene, 2010).

Some authors consider the following practical issues as critically important (Walley and Wright, 2010; WHO, 2008):

- Universal solutions: since there are no universal solutions to the implementation of essential health packages, it implies that solutions to issues of essential health packages should be context-specific, and this requires a great deal of analytical capacity within that setting, and yet the unfortunate reality is that such analytical capacity is in short supply in many resource-poor settings such as in sub-Saharan Africa (Walley and Wright, 2010).

- Measurement problems: whilst in theory, essential health packages are delivered and prioritised in accordance with the disease burden of that particular setting, the reality is that it is not easy to measure disease burden as there is no reliable tool, even though some quantification is required (Walley and Wright, 2010).

- Resource shortfalls: since many resource-poor settings face serious challenges as they are unable to fund even the bare minimum of health services, it would be crucial to involve donors and to have a strong case and motivation to convince donors to fund such essential health packages (Walley and Wright, 2010).

- Maintain current gains: it is possible that some countries may already have had some successes with certain cost-effective health intervention programmes such as immunisation coverage (Walley and Wright, 2010). As such, such successful intervention programmes could not be considered as a priority in terms of the essential health packages, but the issue here is that it would be a mistake that should be guarded against to divert funds from such programmes to interventions that are part of the essential health package (Walley and Wright, 2010).

- Future disease trends: it would be a mistake to merely focus on the current diseases burden and to overlook future diseases trends that may not necessarily be overtly obvious today as such a mistake could prove very costly later on (Walley and Wright, 2010). Given the projection that Africa will see an unprecedented increase in tobacco use over the next few decades, the anti-tobacco legislation in South Africa could prove cost-effective in terms of proactively addressing possible future disease burden related to tobacco smoking (Baleta, 2010).

- Public/political acceptability: involvement of the public and health professionals in in this approach could prove beneficial in terms of their buy-in (Walley and Wright, 2010). It is also critical to bear in mind that in political terms, there has to be a good reason why funds and resources have to be diverted towards this approach to the exclusion of other services (Walley and Wright, 2010). It has to be noted that EHPs can be politically unpopular especially if the argument of holding the government accountable is employed (WHO, 2008). As such, lack of political buy-in could be one of the main limitations of implementing EHPs (WHO, 2008).

- There has to be strong leadership, and it has to be known what service providers will be involved, what will happen if changes in budget allocations are made from other services (Greene, 2010; WHO, 2008).

- Monitoring and evaluation of the EHP: it has to be clear as to who will do the monitoring and how and when the monitoring will be conducted (WHO, 2008).

THE LIMITATIONS AND practical issues of implementing EHPs should be considered to ensure effectiveness of the EHP approach to delivering health services (Mueller et al, 2011). An understanding of the needs and the inherent capacity constraints can clarify the appropriate solution (Sihna and Barry, 2011). As such, what is regarded as evidence-based best practice or innovation that is cost-effective in developed economies may not be applicable to the health-related technologies needed in low- and middle-income countries (Sihna and Barry, 2011).

2.4 Public-private partnerships

WHILST IT IS APPRECIATED that public-private partnerships may create a powerful mechanism for addressing difficult health service delivery problems by leveraging on the strengths of different partners, they also package complex ethical and process-related challenges (Nishtar, 2004). At the level of central administration, a strong central structure, using private-sector expertise, is needed to promote and guide health policy implementation, but the benefits and the imaginative development of policy are weakened by the continuing policy drivers of ideology and off-budget finance, and there is little evidence of a political will to seek a level playing field in the choice between sources of finance (Spackman, 2002).

Public-private partnerships have attracted political attention in South Africa as politicians and industry experts say that partnerships between the public and private sectors may solve the shortage of over 80 000 health professionals including highly skilled and qualified medical laboratory technicians in South Africa (Green, 2013). It is believed that if South Africa wants to deliver a comprehensive and sustainable health care, there is need for resources of both the public and private sectors, as collaborations over a sustained period are likely to succeed (Green, 2013).

However, while theoretically sound, at a practical level it is worth mentioning that public private partnerships can go horribly wrong and cost the state more, as what happened in Britain whereby public private partnerships in the national health system ended up enriching investors rather than benefiting the British public (Fakir, 2011). In fact such a public private partnership was such that the private sector raised the capital to build hospitals and charged the government a monthly fee which has now become an egg on face of the British government (Fakir, 2011).

As such, developing countries such as the Kingdom of Eswatini and the Republic of South Africa are cautioned not to blindly implement public private partnerships if they are not needed (Fakir, 2011). New ventures such as public-private partnerships should be built on need, appropriateness, and lessons on good practice learnt from experience or elsewhere (Widdus, 2001). If governments go ahead or are forced to adopt the public private partnership model, they should be sure that their own capabilities are such that they are able to stand up to the lure and bullying of private sector players, and be able to cap the amount of profits private players can take (Fakir, 2011). In this context, a strong public management capacity is needed to regulate the new market, since without good systems and good information transfer, fragmentation and confusion may ensue (Walley and Wright, 2010).

Whilst there is enthusiasm and potential for gain in terms of efficiency in using public-private partnerships in the delivery of health services for a wider range of health problems, the success of public-private partnerships in this context appears to be mixed (Barr, 2007).

2.5 Healthcare financing

HEALTHCARE FINANCING is one of the critical challenges facing health systems of low- and middle-income countries, and, more recently, healthcare financing features prominently on the global health policy agenda. The challenges are largely brought about by the dilemma of fragile health systems, amid an ever-increasing disease burden, and the prevailing socioeconomic shocks. This is no simple matter, and questions are asked as to how health should be financed, as it is inevitable that the actions needed to attain desired health outcomes must be financed somehow, regardless of the prevailing health systems challenges of those countries.

For example, on 1 June 2018, on the occasion of the official opening of the Central Medical Stores in the Kingdom of Eswatini, it was interesting that the Global Fund's Head of Strategy and Policy, Harley Feldbaum, asserted that the Kingdom of Eswatini should think about innovative ways of financial sustainability for health, as donor funding had flat-lined, and that major increases were unlikely. It is a truism that unless recipient countries urgently take action and come up with mechanisms for sustainable financing for health, the health systems of such countries are in danger of major collapse.

In the context of the vision to eliminate AIDS as a public health issue by 2030, there is some merit in terms of intensification of efforts for the same day initiation of antiretroviral therapy (ART) by international donor agencies, towards achievement of targets, in the short term. However, there is also concern about efficiency and whether the recipient low- and middle-income countries will be able to sustain such efforts beyond the international donor funding. An observation is that there is a general inadequacy of resources in the public health sector of a number of low- and middle-income countries such as in sub-Saharan Africa. In such countries, the supply of therapeutic drugs is not sustainable, which complicates the burden of disease even further, especially among the poor, as the inequities in terms of health access become more skewed in favour of those who can afford, especially in the context of an out-of-pocket payments financing modality. As such, more focus is now on the other financing modalities such as government funding (which is usually not sufficient) and health insurance (of which mandatory health insurance is still non-existent or not fully implemented in many low- and middle-income countries).

With the realisation of the inefficiencies of their respective health systems, and that donor funding is not going to last forever, many recipient low- and middle-income countries, are beginning to seriously assess possible financing mechanisms to improve or replace the existing financing mechanisms. One such mechanism is the basket fund mechanism which involves the pooling of funds from various sources such as government, private sector, and donors to support priorities and ensure adequate resource allocation for agreed upon programme areas (Meghani, Abdulwahab, Privor-Dumm and Wonodi, 2015). While early experiences of basket funds in countries such as Nigeria, show that they enhance availability of funds, accountability and transparency, basket funds should be part of a multi-pronged approach to improve healthcare financing.

There is consensus that equity in healthcare financing should be related to an individual's ability to pay. More specifically, it is accepted that individuals (or families) with different ability to pay should make 'appropriately dissimilar payments' for healthcare with higher income individuals paying more than those with a lower income (referred to as vertical equity). At the same time, it would also be equitable for individuals (or families) with the same ability to pay to contribute the same amount towards their health care costs (referred to as horizontal equity). However, there is less agreement on what is meant by 'appropriately dissimilar payments'. When considering the equity of health care financing, one cannot simply consider who bears the burden of paying for health services; it is equally important to consider who derives the benefit from each source of financing. Thus, it is the combination of the distribution of health care payment burdens relative to ability to pay, and the distribution of health service benefits relative to need, that determine the equity of individual health care financing mechanisms (McIntyre, Gilson, and Mutyambizi, 2005).

2.5.1 Global aid architecture

MANY ECONOMICALLY ADVANCED governments regard official development aid (ODA) as an important tool for promoting economic development, and as an important part of their foreign strategy (Myers, 2016). The United Nations (UN) challenged all economically advanced governments to contribute at least 0.7 per cent of their gross national income to ODA, even though, to date, a few of such countries have met this target (Myers, 2016). As of 2016, the most generous countries in terms of foreign aid were: Sweden (1.41%), United Arab Emirates (1.09%), Norway (1.05%), Luxembourg (0.93%), Denmark (0.85%), Netherlands (0.76%), United Kingdom (0.71%), Finland (0.56%), Turkey (0.54%), Switzerland (0.52%), and Germany (0.52%). The United States of America (USA) came tops in terms of total spend (over $30 billion) through bilateral organisations such as the World Bank or the United Nations (UN).

The global aid architecture which has traditionally consisted of bilateral agencies and non-governmental organisations (NGOs) has undergone major transformations over the past two decades or so. These changes have largely been influenced by increasing pressure to show results of aid; increased demands on official aid budgets, leading to the search for innovative financing mechanisms; changing global conditions such as globalisation, climate change, and persistent political instabilities or conflicts; increased public scrutiny on aid; and the proliferation of new donors, among others. Although global aid programmes have a unique and necessary contribution to make, they are fraught with challenges, such as duplication and overlap with each other, leading to inefficiencies of operation and poor accountability for results (Lele, Sadik and Simmons, 2012).

Coupled with the growing spending on development assistance for health, stimulated by the UN Millennium Development Goals (MDGs) and UN Sustainable Development Goals (SDGs), there has been an interesting transformation of the public health landscape by the emergence of a plethora of vertically funded global health initiatives (Waddington et al, 2009). Some of the major funders of vertical global health initiatives include the Global Alliance for Vaccines and Immunization (GAVI), Global Fund to Fight AIDS, Tuberculosis and Malaria (GFATM), and the United States President's Emergency Plan for AIDS Relief (PEPFAR), among others (Institute for Health Metrics and Evaluation, 2009). It would be interesting to know if this plethora of vertically funded programmes in the health sector is strengthening countries' attempts to improve health or is simply the 'path of least resistance' solutions which avoid some of the difficult complexities of sustainable development.

The influx of so many players into the development assistance arena challenges the overall coordination of the global aid architecture, and, more so, the historic and current dominance of the United States of America (USA). The recent remarkable surge or evolution of China's foreign aid has implications for global aid architecture as it relies on aid principles that are divergent from those of traditional donor countries (Huang and Peiqiang, 2012). In fact, there are ongoing debates about who should call the shots in the global aid architecture. Recommendations are that there should be a global coordinating body or mechanism and standards to ensure equity and fairness both within the donor countries' arena and between the donor countries and recipient countries' arena.

The USA has been a dominant player in global health efforts for more than a century, and, more so, in recent times, where such engagement is sparked by economic, health, and security concerns (Kates, Fischer and Lief, 2009). It is reasoned that, perhaps, the main reason for the USA to assume the de facto first responder for global health crises is due to the absence of effective international institutions (Glassman and Silverman, 2015). The global health engagement of the USA has developed within structure (foreign assistance structure and public health structure), programs and funding (Kates, Fischer and Lief, 2009).

While the foreign assistance structure is predominantly development-oriented and has close links to foreign policy, the public health structure has its roots in disease control and surveillance efforts (Kates, Fischer and Lief, 2009). Most funding and oversight of global health resides within the foreign assistance structure. The main programmatic and funding roles in the USA global health response are played by the State Department and United States Agency for International Development (USAID) play, followed by the Department of Health and Human Services (HHS), and also by a number of other agencies which carry out some global health activities (Kates, Fischer and Lief, 2009).

The USA continues to be the main funder of the global health response, particularly in low- and middle-income countries, even though programming is concentrated in those countries with the heaviest burden of disease, those countries with fragile economies, and those countries where the USA has strategic interests (Kates, Fischer and Lief, 2009). Such funding has significantly increased over time, mainly driven by HIV/AIDS, and, yet, it still constitutes only a small fraction of the overall USA federal budget (Kates, Fischer and Lief, 2009). Most of the global health funding from the USA follows a vertical, disease or problem focused approach, is provided through bilateral channels, primarily through the international affairs budget and through the State Department, USAID, Department of Health and Human Services and its operating divisions (Kates, Fischer and Lief, 2009).

It cannot be denied that initiatives such as the President's Emergency Plan for AIDS (PEPFAR) and the President's Malaria Initiative have been effective to a certain degree (Glassman and Silverman, 2015). However, it is argued that the USA's global health response follows outmoded and inefficient models which fail to reflect emerging challenges, threats, and financial constraints (Glassman and Silverman, 2015). The immediate quick responses in committing funds to fight emerging and remerging diseases such as Ebola is commendable, but, committing funds without strengthening systems is a problem, and unsustainable. As she was speaking to USA law makers in a congressional hearing in May 2018, it was interesting to see the USA Global AIDS Coordinator Deborah Birx questioning the effectiveness of the US$3 billion spent on supply chain since 2009 and also made reference to glitches in the USAD's US$9.5 billion project (Henry J Kaiser Family Foundation, 2018). As such, it is recommended that the USA should prioritise and strengthen global health leadership and accountability, health and economic impact, partnerships for sustainable health investment, and drive reforms at related multilateral organisations such as WHO, GAVI, and Global Fund (Glassman and Silverman, 2015).

Much as the USA is the largest donor to global health efforts, the USA has its own domestic health policy and programme challenges. In fact, the USA is ranked as the worst performing health system out of a total of eleven richest countries, particularly in the context of measures of access, affordability, health outcomes, and equality between the rich and the poor (Khazan, 2017). The USA health policy challenges include lack of cross-party political consensus, lack of stringent spending controls, poor accountability and oversight of insurance companies, and prohibition of the creation of institutes for the assessment of the cost-effectiveness of pharmaceuticals, health services and technologies in the context of the implementation of the Patient Protection and Affordable Care Act – commonly known as the Affordable Care Act (ACA) or Obamacare (Rice et al, 2014).

The plethora of vertically funded programmes has had some positive effects in the sense that this has brought much needed resources to help contribute towards the strengthening of health systems especially in low- and middle-income countries. Judging from what has been observed in the Southern African Development Community (SADC), those vertically funded programmes concerned with HIV/AIDS have not only increased access and uptake of HIV/AIDS services, but they have also resulted in a broader use of HIV-specific resources for the improvement of primary health care in general. Merson, Black and Mills (2012) highlight that vertically funded HIV/AIDS-specific programmes have resulted in the upgrade of health facilities and infrastructure, training and empowerment of health care workers, and an overall improved primary health care service in countries such as Haiti and Rwanda, among others.

On the other hand, the vertically funded programmes in the health sector have also had negative effects on countries' attempts to strengthen health systems. Much as the HIV/AIDS specific vertically funded programmes have increased access to health care facilities, this has also increased the pressure on the health care workforce in the public sector, to such an extent that the increased workload has somewhat demoralised the poorly paid health care workforce, especially in disease burdened countries. Such programmes have been costly in the sense that they tend to concentrate on a particular area of diseases expertise and neglect others, and that such programmes can be difficult to establish, monitor, or to even assess their effectiveness (Merson, Black and Mills, 2012).

According to Travis et al (2004), the disease-based approach takes a unilateral and narrow view to health provision in the sense that it employs systems such as planning, management and financing that are separate from other systems, while the system/sector based approach is horizontal and takes an integrative view to health provision, and uses existing health system structures. The vertical approach focuses on fighting one disease at a time whereas the horizontal or sector-wide approach (SWAp) invests sector-wide to make health systems work to administer prevention and treatment for all diseases (Easterly and Frechi, 2010).

Merson, Black and Mills (2012) define a SWAp as an approach to a locally-owned programme for a coherent sector in a comprehensive and coordinated manner, moving toward the use of country systems. Sector wide approaches have been perceived as being the answer to competition and duplication, as well as improving health system equity and efficiency by ensuring a more effective way of managing resources in line with national needs and priorities (McIntyre, 2007).

The vertical disease-based approach has minimal impact because of the involvement of varied players and activities having competing, overlapping, and, only rarely, shared approaches (Birn, Pillay and Holtz, 2009). This results not only in fragmentation of efforts but also in competition and duplication because of poor coordination.

The UN Millennium Development Goals (MDGs) somewhat created a strong emphasis on specific disease initiatives, such as the HIV/AIDS, Malaria and Tuberculosis initiatives, with the assumption that if the goals of such specific initiatives were achieved, the health system would also be strengthened. The irony though is that such specific disease initiatives appear to overlook the fact that many low- and middle-income countries have low capacity to deliver, and therefore the specific disease initiatives may end up weakening the already weak health systems (Travis et al, 2004).

From the perspective of a failing disease-focused TB or Malaria programme to a sector-wide approach (SWAp), there would be a need to ensure that there is coordination, reduction of duplication of service provision and development of a single, sustainable coherent vision that is led by the recipient government with reliance on local knowledge and methodologies (Birn, Pillay and Holtz, 2009).

It is encouraging though, that there has been growing recognition of the limitations of the disease-based or vertical approach, lately. As a result, there has been a move towards an integrative sector-based approach being adopted in a number of settings in a number of low- and middle-income countries. According to Hutton and Tanner (2004), the advantage of a system- or sector-based approach is that it is comprehensive and allows the synchronisation of planning and pooling of resources. This can enhance equitable access to health care services and the inequalities or differences in health status experienced by the local population will be addressed, but the disadvantage is that it is not that easy to monitor and measure a system-based approach (Travis et al, 2004).

Proponents of the disease-based approach such as the HIV/AIDS programme claim that it is advantageous because it is cost-effective, more focused and the results are measurable (Birn, Pillay and Holtz, 2009). The disadvantage is that it fails to consider the root causes or the complexities of the constraints beyond specific disease programmes such as public sector employment rules, and sustainability issues (Travis et al, 2004).

It is of concern that so much intensification of efforts and investment is channelled towards HIV treatment, and not so much on prevention of new infections. The opportunity cost is also an issue, as there seems to be so much focus on HIV and AIDS, and not so much on other major public health issues such as the emerging epidemic of a plethora of chronic non-communicable diseases and co-morbidities crippling the health system. It is also of concern that there is poor or lack of integration of HIV prevention interventions as well as poor or lack of continuum between HIV prevention, treatment and care at both coordination and implementation levels of the HIV and AIDS response. The vertical focus on public health issues is inefficient and unsustainable.

A disease-based approach appears to worsen health inequities and inequalities in the local population, while a system- or sector-based approach appears to address this issue. On the other hand, it is argued that SWAps are a good idea in theory but a disaster in practice, in the sense that SWAps focus on the process of coordinating aid delivery, which has become an end in itself, obscuring the need to actually increase successful treatment and decrease deaths (Easterly and Frechi, 2010). For example, it is reported that only a few of the World Bank SWAp projects in sub-Saharan Africa from 2001 to 2008 have shown successful health outcomes. In fact, it was only in Tanzania where a SWAp might have been linked to an actual health outcome: higher rates of TB treatment success (Easterly and Frechi, 2010).

To move from a failing disease-focused TB or Malaria programme to a SWAp, there would be a need to create incentives to focus on results, not the process, drastically increase transparency of project information and evaluation, and do independent programme evaluation (Easterly and Frechi, 2010).

While the limitations of disease-focused approaches have been highlighted by a number of studies, sector-wide approaches (SWAps) have offered some promise in terms of harmonising aid and assimilating various sectors and role players with the goal of strengthening health systems, but on the other hand the overall success and sustainability of SWAps is in doubt (Wiley and Wright, 2010). As such, it would be crucial to re-evaluate systems and structures in healthcare provision.

An evaluation in 2010 of health SWAps in six countries (Bangladesh, Ghana, Kyrgyzstan, Malawi, Nepal, and Tanzania) produced mixed results (Merson, Black and Mills, 2012). On the one hand, the SWAps had been successful in putting in place tools and processes for improved sector coordination and oversight, and had made headway in improving the harmonisation and alignment of development assistance (Merson, Black and Mills, 2012). On the other hand, SWAps had been only modestly successful in achieving improvements in the efficiency of resource utilisation, the ability to focus on results, and the enforcement of sector-wide accountabilities (of government and donors) (Merson, Black and Mills, 2012). The majority of completed programmes of work had made only modest progress in achieving their nationally set development objectives (Merson, Black and Mills, 2012).

Some authors observe that the difficulty with evaluating SWAps is that sustained reforms take time and that in SWAps there is no universal standard to determine the point at which tangible benefits to population health can be demonstrated (Hutton and Tanner, 2004). It is therefore suggested that accurate and comprehensive monitoring programmes tailored to specific system contexts must be set up, preferably based on demographic surveillance systems (Hutton and Tanner, 2004).

Walley and Wright (2010) argue that the emergence of large disease-specific global funds such as the Global Fund for AIDS, Tuberculosis and Malaria threatens to re-fragment health systems which were integrating funding and service provision. It has been observed that the Global Fund has somewhat created a dependency in a number of low- and middle-income countries, particularly, in sub-Saharan African. This appears to leave these recipient countries in a dilemma, because on the one hand, these countries have the intention to implement SWAps, but on the other hand the major donors do not want to get involved with the SWAps, and this undermines the SWAps' effectiveness.

Moving from a failing disease-focused program to a SWAp may seem attractive, but SWAps have their own inherent challenges largely because they vary in different contexts, and therefore very difficult to monitor and evaluate in terms of their population health impact. Both the disease-specific approach and the sector-wide approach (SWAp) have a role to play in reducing inequalities. However, the context of low- and middle-income countries poses many challenges, unless the more fundamental causes of poverty and inequity are addressed, as many of the poorest countries are trapped in a cycle of debt, unfair trade restrictions and undemocratic international policymaking that protects the wealthy at the expense of the poor (Poore, 2004).

These challenges are exacerbated by the tendency for international donors to react or respond to a crisis situation such as the burden of HIV/AIDS, Malaria and Tuberculosis in low- and middle-income countries such as in the sub-Saharan Africa. The reactionary tendency or crisis mentality stimulated by effective advocacy programmes puts more emphasis on the treatment of communicable diseases such as Tuberculosis and in the process inadvertently compromises or undermines the long-term view of sustainability and strengthening the health system.

It is interesting that the South African government has committed to employing a SWAp or an integrated health system. However, the dominance of international donors and global health initiatives on communicable diseases such as the Global Fund to fight AIDS, Tuberculosis and Malaria has made this look more like a disease-focused approach, as there does not seem to be an agreed-upon strategy by all role players. Chansa et al (2008) observe that despite the strong commitment to implement SWAp in Zambia, the envisaged efficiency improvements do not seem to have been attained, possibly because the SWAp has not been fully developed or that not all parties have completely embraced it. This calls for urgent evaluation of the approach. For example, the Department for International Development (DFID) agreed with the Government of Malawi to commission an impact evaluation of SWAp, and this evaluation was done in phases (Pearson, 2010).

Even if there is a move from a collapsing disease-focused approach to a SWAp or an integrated approach, the bottom line is that if the fundamental causes of poverty and inequity are not addressed, such an approach is bound to fail, and particularly so if the long-term view is ignored or overlooked. Clearly, a SWAp may not be appropriate in all cases – particularly where there is no agreed-upon strategy, where demand for this approach is not initiated by the government, where opinions differ between a government and donors (Lele, Ridker and Upadhyay, 2005).

⸻ ◉ ⸻

2.6 Monitoring performance

IT IS A PAINFUL REALITY that most countries have an inability to generate the data needed to monitor performance in health care delivery (AbouZahr and Boerma, 2005).

Given the increasing importance of performance indicators in health policy, the availability of quality data is crucial, but bearing in mind the potential problems associated with obtaining and utilising the data (Freeman, 2002). Some of the major problems include the potential to undermine the conditions required for quality improvement, perverse incentives and the difficulty of using data to promote change (Freeman, 2002). AbouZahr and Boerma (2005) observe that international donors in health are largely responsible for the problems, having prioritised urgent needs for data over longer-term country capacity-building.

There is a lot that is happening to try and make quality data available in many low- and middle-income countries, and there are many different actors involved at different levels of the health care system, and so many different sources of data and the use of different indicators, thus creating more confusion for decision-makers (Mate et al, 2009). As such, there is an urgent need for a framework for integrating, validating, analysing, and disseminating the fragmentary and at times contradictory information that is available (Lopez et al, 2006).

Health surveillance and information systems have also been implemented to generate, analyse and disseminate such data (Mate et al, 2009). The reality is that health information systems rarely function systematically as they are products of historical, social and economic forces, and they are complex, fragmented and unresponsive to needs (AbouZahr and Boerma, 2005).

Some policymakers may think that investing more money will solve the problem, however the reality is that money alone is likely to be insufficient unless accompanied by sustained support to country systems development coupled with greater donor accountability and allocation of resources AbouZahr and Boerma (2005).

The monitoring of performance indicators in health performance management systems has heavily influenced debate over their value (Freeman, 2002). Whilst the importance of the availability of quality data cannot be denied, the main challenge is the capacity to apply it, and this creates more confusion, as policy-makers end up taking the data at face value and taking decisions that are not applicable or appropriate to the particular context of the setting.

Given the uniqueness of different settings, should different countries have their own set of indicators to monitor performance of health care delivery? In contrast, Lewis and Pettersson (2005) propose performance indicators that offer the potential for comparable measures as useful tools for cross-country comparisons and for tracking relative health performance.

Whether cross-cutting or country-specific indicators are used, the crucial thing is to ensure that there is good governance, since good governance is central to enhancing performance in health care delivery (Lewis and Pettersson, 2005). Crucial to high performance are standards, information, incentives and accountability (Lewis and Pettersson, 2005).

However, it has to be borne in mind that ensuring good governance is not always easy especially where there is rapid transformation of jurisdictions such as in post-apartheid South Africa (Coovadia et al, 2009). Given the restructuring of jurisdictions in South Africa, the public health system has also been transformed, but failures in leadership and stewardship and weak management have led to inadequate implementation of what are often good policies (Coovadia et al. 2009). As such, inadequate implementation of good policies appears to compromise efforts towards good governance such as in health care service delivery, thereby making it seem as if good-governance is done in a vacuum (Taylor, 2000).

Much as the importance of a context-specific approach in terms of each country having its own set of indicators is valid, good governance should also be approached from a deeper angle as it is not that obviously clear in different settings. In fact, some authors observe that the good governance agenda is unrealistically long and growing longer over time, because there is little guidance about what is essential and what is not, what should come first and what should follow, what can be achieved in the short term and what can only be achieved over the long term, what is feasible and what is not (Grindle, 2004). If more attention is given to sorting out these questions, "good enough governance" may become a more realistic goal for many countries faced with the goal of reducing poverty. Working toward good enough governance means accepting a more nuanced understanding of the evolution of institutions and government capabilities; being explicit about trade-offs and priorities in a world in which all good things cannot be pursued at once; learning about what is working rather than focusing solely on governance gaps; taking the role of government in poverty alleviation seriously; and grounding action in the contextual realities of each country (Grindle, 2004).

The distinctive good governance issues and challenges that must be faced in health care delivery are often neither fully recognised nor addressed, yet, governance can serve as a critical facilitator of, or a barrier to, achieving high performance in health care delivery (Alexander, Zuckerman and Pointer, 1995).

References

AbouZahr, C. & Boerma, T. (2005) 'Health information systems: the foundations of public health', *Bulletin of the World Health Organization*, 83, pp. 578-583.

Alexander, J.A., Zuckerman, H.S. & Pointer, D. (1995) 'The challenges of governing integrated health care systems', *Health Care Management Review*, 20 (4), pp. 69-81.

Alva, S., Kleinau, E., Pomeroy, A. & Rowan, K. (2009). *Measuring the impact of health systems strengthening: a review of the literature*. US Agency for International Development.

Baleta, A. (2010) 'Africa's struggle to be smoke free', *The Lancet*, 375 (9709), pp. 107-108.

Barr, D.A. (2007) 'A research protocol to evaluate the effectiveness of public-private partnerships as a means to improve health and welfare systems worldwide', *American Journal of Public Health*, 97 (1), pp. 19-25.

Bheekie, A., Adonis, T. & Daniels, P. (2009) 'Contextualising undergraduate pharmacy training in service-learning at the university of the Western Cape', *Education as Change*, 11 (3), pp. 157-167.

Birn, A. & Richter, J. (2017) U.S. *Philanthrocapitalism and the Global Health Agenda: The Rockefeller and Gates Foundations, Past and Present*. Global Policy Forum: New York.

Birn, A., Pillay, Y. & Holtz, T.H. (2009) *Textbook of international health: global health in a dynamic world*. New York: Oxford.

Birx, D., de Souza, M. & Nkengasong, N. (2009) 'Laboratory challenges in the scaling up of HIV, TB, and Malaria programs', *American Journal of Pathology*, 131, pp. 849-851.

Coovadia, H., Jeukes, R., Baron, P., Sanders, D. & McIntyre, D. (2009) 'The health and health system of South Africa: historical roots of current public health challenges', *Lancet*, 374, pp. 817-834.

Dacombe, R.E., Squire, S.B., Ramsay, A.R.C, Banda, H.T. & Bates, I. (2006) 'Essential medical laboratory services: their role in delivering equitable health care in Malawi', *Malawi Medical Journal*, 18 (2), pp. 77-79.

Danish Ministry of Foreign Affairs. (2007). *Controversies in health care financing: perspectives and debate.* Special Session at the 6th Congress of iHEA.

Department for International Development (DFID) (2006) *How to note: How to provide technical cooperation personnel*, June.

Derua, Y., Ishengoma, D.R.S., Rwegoshora, R.T., Tenu, F., Massaga, J.J., Mboera, L.E.G. & Magesa, S.M. (2011) 'Users' and health service providers' perception on quality of laboratory malaria diagnosis in Tanzania', *Malaria Journal*, 10:78.

Dewhusrt, M., Guthridge, M. & Mohr, E. (2009) Motivating people: getting beyond money. *McKinsey Quarterly*, November.

Ditlopo, P., Blaauw, D., Rispel, L.C., Thomas, S. & Bidwell, P. (2013) 'Policy implementation and financial incentives for nurses in South Africa: a case study on the occupation-specific dispensation', *Global Health Action*, 6 (10).

Ditlopo, P., Blaauw, D., Bidwell, P. & Thomas, S. (2011) 'Analysing the implementation of the rural allowance in hospitals in North West Province, South Africa', *Public Health Policy*, 32 (Suppl).

Drummond, M.F., Schwartz, J.S., Johnsson, B., Luce, B.R., Neumann, P.J., Siebert, U. & Sullivan, S.D. (2008) 'Key principles for the improved conduct of health technology assessments for resource allocation decisions', *International Journal of Technology Assessment in Health Care*, 24 (3), pp. 244-258.

Dwyer, J. & Wilhelmsen, S. (n.d.). *Leadership and management.*

Easterly, W. & Frechi, L. (2010) *The World Bank's "horizontal" approach to health falls horizontal.*

Eghan, K. (2018) Strong pharmaceutical systems are crucial to attaining UHC. *Health systems strengthening,* May 24, 2018.

Ensor, T., Dave-Sen, P., Ali, L., Hossain, A., Begum, S.A. & Moral, H. (2002) 'Do essential service packages benefit the poor? Preliminary evidence from Bangladesh', *Health Policy and Planning*, 17 (3), pp. 247-256.

Fakir, (2011) 'Lessons for South Africa from England's messy public-private partnerships', *The South African Civil Society Information Service*, 10 February.

Feiring, B. (2003) *Indigenous peoples and poverty: the cases of Bolivia, Guatemala, Honduras and Nicaragua.* Minority Rights Group International.

Forster, A.J., Turnbull, J., McGuire, S., Ho, M.L. & Worthington, J.R. (2011) 'Improving patient safety and physician accountability using the hospital credentialing process', *Open Medicine*, 5 (2).

Frenk, J., Chen, L., Bhutta, Z.A., Cohen, J., Crisp, N., Evans, T., Fineberg, H., Garcia, P., Ke, Y., Kelley, P., Kistnasamy, B., Meleis, A., Naylor, D., Pablos-Mendez, A., Reddy, S., Scrimshaw, S., Sepulveda, J., Serwadda, D. & Zurayk, H. (2010) 'Health professionals for a new century: transforming education to strengthen health systems in an interdependent world', *The Lancet*, 376, pp. 1923-1958.

Frenk, J. (2006) 'Bridging the divide: global lessons from evidence-based health policy in Mexico', *Lancet*, 368, pp. 954-961.

Fried, L.P., Piot, P., Frenk, J.J., Flahault, A. & Parker, R. (2012). Global public health leadership for the twenty-first century: towards improved health of all populations. *Global Public Health*, 7(S1), S5-S15.

Friedland, G., Harris, A. & Coetzee, D. (2007) 'Implementation issues in Tuberculosis/HIV program collaboration and integration: 3 case studies', The *Journal of Infectious Diseases*, 196 (suppl. 1), pp. S114-S123.

Glassman, A. & Silverman, R. (2016) Restructuring US global health programs to respond to new challenges and missed opportunities. *The White House and the World.*

Go Molecular (n.d.) *Sample transport in Uganda: a network for efficiency.*

Gostin, L. & Friedman, E.A. (2014). Ebola: a crisis in global health leadership. *The Lancet*, 384, 1323-1325. Retrieved May 10, 2015 from http://www.thelencet.com

Green, A. (2013) 'Public private partnerships may answer doctor shortage', *Mail & Guardian*, 19 August.

Greene, J.A. (2010) 'When did medicines become essential?', *Bulletin of the World Health Organization*, 88 (7), pp. 483.

Grindle, M.S. (2004) 'Good governance: poverty reduction and reform in developing countries', *Governance*, 17 (4), pp. 525-548.

Haines, A., Kuruvilla, S., Borchert, M. (2004) 'Bridging the implementation gap between knowledge and action for health', *Bulletin of the World Health Organization*, 82, pp. 724-732.

Heading, G. (2009). *Strategic leadership, culture and change in health services.* Alexandria: Cancer Institute NSW.

Henry J Kaiser Family Foundation (2018) *Kaiser Daily Global Health Policy Report*, May 21, 2018.

Huang, M. & Peiqiang, R. (2012) *China's foreign aid and its role in the international aid architecture.* Emerging economies and global policies, pp. 75-78

Johnson, J.A. & Stoskopf, C. (2010). *Comparative health systems: global perspectives.* New York: Jones & Bartlett.

Jooste, K. (2009) *Leadership in health services management.* Lansdowne: Juta

Kates, J., Fischer, J. & Lief, E. (2009) The U.S. government's global health policy architecture: structure, programs, and funding. The Henry J. Kaiser Family Foundation. *U.S. Global health Policy.*

Kelley, E.T., Arispe, I. & Holmes, J. (2006). Beyond the initial indicators: lessons from the OECD health care quality indicators project and the US national healthcare quality report. *International Journal for Quality in Health Care*, 45-51.

Khazan. O. (2017) What's actually wrong with the U.S. health system. *The Atlantic*.

Kiyaga, C., Sendagire, H., Joseph, E MConnll, I., Grosz, J., Narayan, V., Esiru, G., Elyanu, P., Akol, Z., Kirungi, W., Musingizi, & Opio, A. (2013) 'Uganda's new national laboratory sample transport system: a successful model for improving access to diagnostic services for early infant HIV diagnosis and other programs', *PLoS One*, 8 (11): e78609.

Kumar, S., Kumar, N. & Vivekadhish, S. (2016) Millennium Development Goals (MDGs) to Sustainable Development Goals (SDGs): addressing unfinished agenda and strengthening sustainable development and partnership. *Indian Journal of Community Medicine*, 41(1): 1-4.

Kumar, A. & Ozdamar, L. (2004). International comparison of health care systems. *International Journal of the Computer, The Internet and Management*, 12(3), 81-95.

Lele, Sadik and Simmons, (2012) *Changing Aid Architecture: can global initiatives eradicate poverty?* [Online].

Lewis, M. & Pettersson, G. (2009) 'Governance in health care delivery: raising performance', *Policy Research Working Paper*, 5074. Washington DC: World Bank.

Lewis, M. & Pettersson, G. (2005) *Governance in health care delivery: raising performance.* World Health Workforce Alliance, Geneva: World Health Organization.

Lopez, A., Mathers, C., Ezzati, M., Jamison, D.T. & Murray, C.J.L. (2006) 'Global and regional burden of disease and risk factors, 2001: systematic analysis of population health data', *The Lancet*, 367 (9524), pp. 1747-1757.

Magowe, M.K., Lediwe, J.H., Kasvosve, I., Martin, R., Thankane, K. & Semo, B. (2014) 'An innovative educational approach to professional development of medical laboratory scientists in Botswana', *Advances in Medical Education and Practice*, 4 (5), pp. 73-81.

Mate, K.S., Bennett, B., Mphatswe, W., Parker, P. & Rollins, N. (2009) 'Challenges for routine health system data management in a large public programme to prevent mother-to-child transmission in South Africa', *PLoS ONE*, 4 (5): e5483.

McIntyre, D. (2007) *Learning from experience: health care financing in low- and middle-income countries.* Global Forum for Health Research, Geneva.

Merson, M.H., Black, R.E. & Mills, A.J. (2012) *Global health: diseases, programs, systems, and policies.* London: Jones & Bartlett.

Ministry of Foreign Affairs of Denmark (2013) *Denmark-Bolivia Country Policy Paper 2013-2018.* Copenhagen. www.danida-publikationer.dk

Mitton, C., Adair, C.E., McKenzie, E., Patten, S.B. & Perry, B.W. (2007) 'Knowledge transfer and exchange: review and synthesis of the literature', *The Milbank Quarterly*, 85 (4), pp. 729-768.

Montegut, A.J. (2007). To achieve "health for all" we must shift the world's paradigm to "primary care access for all". *Journal of the American Board of Family Medicine.*

Mossman, K., McGahan, A., Mitchell, W. & Bhattacharyya, O. (2014) 'Evaluating high-tech health approaches in low-income countries', *Stanford Social Innovation Review*, 11 February.

Mullan, F., Frehywat, S., Omaswa, F., et al. (2011) 'Medical schools in sub-Saharan Africa', *The Lancet*, 377, pp. 1113-1121.

Mueller, D.H., Lungu, D., Acharya, A. & Palmer, N. (2011) 'Constraints to implementing the essential health package in Malawi', *Public Library of Sciences*, e20741.

Myers, J. (2016) *Foreign aid: these countries are the most generous.* World Economic Forum.

Ndihokubwayo, J.B., Kasolo, F., Yahaya, A.M. & Mwenda, J. (2010) 'Strengthening public health laboratories in the WHO Africa region: a critical need for disease control', *The African Health Monitor*, (12), April-June.

Nishtar, S., Niinisto, S., Vazquez, T. et al. (2018) Time to deliver: report of the WHO Independent High-level Commission on NCDs. *Lancet*, 6736(18):31258-3.

Nishtar, S. (2004) 'Public-private 'partnerships' in health – a global call to action', *Health Research Policy and Systems*, 2:5.

Opio, A., Wafula, W., Amone, J., Kajumbula, H., Nkengasong, J.N. (2010). Country leadership and policy are critical factors for implementing laboratory accreditation in developing countries. *American Journal of Clinical Pathology*, 134, 381-387.

Pruitt, S.D. & Epping-Jordan, J. (2005) 'Preparing the 21st century global healthcare workforce', *The Lancet*, 330, pp. 637-639.

Quick, J.D. (2011) *Strong leadership, management, and governance practices improve health impact.*

Ruff, B., Mzimba, M., Hendrie, S. & Broomberg, J. (2011) 'Reflections on health-care reforms in South Africa', *Journal of Public Health Policy*, 32, pp. s184-s192.

Smith, P.C. & Papanicolas, I. (2012). *Health system performance comparison: an agenda for policy, information and research.* Copenhagen: World Health Organization.

Sullivan, T.M., Limaye, R.J., Mitchell, V., D'Adamo, M. & Baquef,, Z. (2015) Levaraging the power of knowledge management to transform global health and development, *Global Health: Science and Practice*, 3(2), pp. 150-162.

Taylor, D.W. (2000) 'Facts, myths and monsters: understanding the principles of good governance', *The International Journal of Public Sector Management*, 13 (2), pp. 108-124.

USAID (2012) *The intersection of knowledge management and health systems strengthening: implications from the Malawi Knowledge for Health Demonstration Project* [Online].

Victora, C.G., Hanson, K., Bryce, J. & Vaughan, J.P. (2004) 'Achieving universal coverage with health interventions', *Lancet*, 364, pp. 1541-1548.

Walley, J. & Wright, J. (2010) *Public health: an action guide to improving health*. New York: Oxford.

Waddington, C., Hadi, Y., Pearson, M., Alebachew, A., Eldon, J., James, J., Khan, M.S. & Varghese, B. (2009) *Global aid architecture and the health millennium development goals*. Oslo: Norwegian Agency for Development Cooperation.

Widdus, R. (2001) 'Public-private partnerships for health: their main targets, their diversity, and their future directions', *Bulletin of the World Health Organization*, 79, pp. 713-720.

Woltring, C., Constantine, W. & Schwarte, L. (2003). Does leadership training make a difference? The CDC/UC public health leadership institute. *Journal of Public Health Management & Practice*, 9(2), 103-122.

World Health Organization (WHO) (2008) 'Essential health packages: what are they for? what do they change?', *WHO Service Delivery Seminar Series, DRAFT Technical Brief No. 2*, July.

World Health Organization (WHO). (2007). *Building leadership and management capacity in health*. Geneva: World Health Organization.

World Health Organization (WHO) (2007) *Everybody's business: strengthening health systems to improve health outcomes: WHO's framework for action*. Geneva: World Health Organization.

World Health Organization (2006) *Bridging the "know-do" gap meeting on knowledge translation in global health*.

World Health Organization (WHO) (2006) World health report 2006: working together for health. Geneva. *World Health Organization*.

World Health Organization (WHO) (2000) *Health systems: improving performance*. Geneva: World Health Organization.

World Health Professions Alliance (WHPA) (2007) *A core competency framework for international health consultants*. Geneva: World Health Professions Alliance.

Chapter 3
Engineering Better Health and Care

Abstract
This chapter presents an overview and impact of engineering better health and care. Some of the key highlights of this chapter are that a new paradigm is needed for the design and integration of technology within the healthcare setting to achieve the advantages of interoperability. This new paradigm is needed because today's medical systems are effectively closed proprietary systems that severely curtail the ability to extract data and information. Successful systems engineering delivery process in healthcare should focus on defining stakeholder needs and required functionality early in the development cycle. Clinical engineering departments should continue striving to keep up with the rapid future technology demands and to increase the awareness of hospital administrations to support their continuous staff development programmes. More meticulous planning for stocking a reasonable number of spare parts, especially for vital equipment, in order to minimise equipment down time, should be implemented. Careful selection of equipment for purchase with an emphasis on after sale service is a necessity, to avoid withdrawal or lack of service support.

Key words:

KEY WORDS: Healthcare systems engineering, technology, health, medicine, clinical engineering, technology, health, medicine, analysis, cultural, social, knowledge, technical, regulatory, policy, financial, economic.

3.1 Introduction

MODERN MEDICINE DEFINES the cutting edge in most fields of clinical research, training, and practice worldwide, and manufacturers of drugs, medical devices, and medical equipment are among the most innovative and competitive areas. In large part, many countries, especially high-income countries have achieved primacy in these areas by focusing public and private resources on research in the life and physical sciences and on the engineering of devices, instruments, and equipment to serve individual patients.

At the same time, very little technical talent or material resources have been devoted to improving or optimising the operations or measuring the quality and productivity of the overall healthcare system. The costs of this collective inattention and the failure to take advantage of the tools, knowledge, and infrastructure that have yielded quality and productivity revolutions in many other sectors have been enormous.

One need only note that hundreds of thousands of people die, and millions of patients suffer injuries each year as a result of broken health care processes and system failures; and an estimated thirty percent of every dollar spent on health care, is spent on costs associated with "overuse, underuse, or poor communication, and inefficiency" (Lawrence,). Health care costs have been rising at double digit-rates – roughly three times the rate of inflation, claiming a growing share of every person's income, inflicting economic hardships on many, and decreasing access to care.

As such, healthcare organisations around the world are transforming themselves into more efficient, coordinated and user-centred systems. This tendency implies that more integrated interoperable and ubiquitous healthcare services, a greater and easier access to health records and related information, and to engage patients in their own healthcare. With this purpose, and through advocacy, the information and communication technology should play a more central role in achieving efficient and accessible healthcare systems that should fulfil and address diverse and frequently overlooked aspects of healthcare systems. One could paraphrase George Clemenceau (1841-1929) by saying that perhaps health is too important to be left only to doctors, data analytics enables getting objective data and information and well- grounded decision making (Fernandez and Pallis, 2014).

3.2 Health Systems Engineering

IN ESSENCE, SIMILAR to the engineering discipline of manufacturing systems engineering, the requirements of systems thinking in healthcare improvement can be summarised in terms of three key principles: systems perspective of health processes, structured problem-solving, and the closed-loop of continuous improvement. Despite their diversity, all systems have some characteristics in common. As a result, systems concepts have been applied in many of the fundamental fields of science and most branches of engineering and management.

However, until recently, the traditional approach to healthcare improvement has been based on specialised and isolated segments. Very rarely was a healthcare process viewed from a systems perspective as an integrated combination of processes, equipment, people, organisational structures, information flows, control systems and computers, designed and operated in order properly to support a coherent goal. The key issues of attaining excellence rely on the adoption of the appropriate methodology, as well as technology.

Healthcare systems engineering is an area of research in healthcare delivery science that examines system and process design. Researchers in health systems engineering seek to increase efficiency, reduce errors, and improve access and overall quality of healthcare. The major areas in healthcare systems engineering are: human factors engineering and systems integration; and information and decision engineering (Mayo Clinic, 2021).

In human factors engineering and systems integration, scientists use ergonomics and organisation science to identify and correct incompatibilities among people, technology and work environments. Research focus on improving technologies and systems to be as effective as possible within the physical and psychological limitations of humans (Mayo Clinic, 2021).

Information and decision engineering is based on data-driven and mathematical sciences, including operations research, statistics, informatics, management and computational sciences. Scientists focus on quantitative evaluation and modelling of processes and systems of healthcare. They work to identify the best possible ways to deliver care and to build evidence base for data-driven decision-making (Mayo Clinic, 2021).

Healthcare Systems Engineering entails the application of engineering, science, management, and technological innovation to healthcare systems improvement. The myriad of challenges and opportunities that come with rapid technological innovations in healthcare and medicine, warrant an urgent need to apply systems engineering techniques and skills to solve issues pertaining to healthcare service quality, patient safety, and healthcare cost, as means to improve healthcare systems performance. Health systems engineering can solve healthcare problems that no one else can.

Systems engineering tools have been used in a wide variety of applications to achieve major improvements in the quality, efficiency, safety, and/or custom-centredness of processes, products, and services in a wide range of manufacturing and service industries. The health care sector as a whole has been very slow to embrace them, however, even though they have been shown to yield valuable returns to the small but growing number of health care organisations and clinicians that have applied them (Murray and Berwick, 2003).

Statistical process controls, queuing theory, quality function deployment, failure-mode effects analysis, modelling and simulation, human-factors engineering have been adapted to applications in health care delivery and used tactically by clinicians, care teams, and administrators in large health care organisations to improve the performance of discrete care processes, units, and departments.

However, the strategic use of these and more information technology-intensive tools from the fields of enterprise and supply-chain management, financial engineering and risk analysis, and knowledge discovery in databases has been limited. With some adaptations, these tools could be used to measure, characterise, and optimise performance at higher levels of the health care system (such as, individual health care organisations, regional care systems, the public health system, the health research enterprise, and so forth). The most promising systems engineering tools and areas of associated research are listed below (Reid et al, 2005):

- **System-design tools**
    - Concurrent engineering and quality function deployment
    - Human-factors tools
    - Failure mode effects analysis
- **Systems-analysis tools**
    - Modelling and simulation
        - Queuing methods
        - Discrete-event simulation
    - Enterprise-management tools
        - Supply-chain management
        - Game theory and contracts
        - Systems dynamics models

- Productivity measuring and monitoring
  - Financial engineering and risk analysis tools
    - Stochastic analysis
    - Value-at-risk
    - Optimisation tools for individual decision-making
    - Distributed decision-making: market models and agency theory
  - Knowledge discovery in databases
    - Data mining
    - Predictive modelling
    - Neural networks
- **Systems-control tools**
  - Statistical process control
  - Scheduling

Although data and associated information technology needs do not present significant technical or cost barriers to the tactical application of systems engineering tools, there are significant structural, technical, and cost-related barriers at the organisational, multi-organisational, and environmental levels to the strategic implementation of systems tools.

3.2.1 Impact of Healthcare Systems Engineering

THE IMPACT OF HEALTHCARE systems engineering on the healthcare and medical ecosystem encompasses the following categories: clinical effectiveness; healthcare provider aspects; patient safety and security; economic and financial aspects; organisational aspects, socio-cultural aspects; legal and regulatory aspects.

3.2.1.1 Clinical effectiveness

APPLICATION OF ENGINEERING systems models in healthcare and medicine enables improvement to clinician knowledge (Royal Academy of Engineering, 2017).

Healthcare systems engineering can enable significant opportunities to answer questions in the healthcare system. In terms of healthcare operations management, healthcare systems engineering can provide answers on how surgeries in an outpatient procedure centre be scheduled in order to minimise overtime and waiting time for the patient; the best strategy to schedule outpatient appointments in order to reduce overtime and no-shows; how to reduce what can be considered waste in the healthcare system; when should the emergency department decide to go on diversion and how waiting times can be reduced; the best staffing level for every department, everyday; levels of medical supplies needed; and on how information and communication technology in the healthcare system be implemented (Fowler et al, 2011).

In terms of socio-technical systems analysis, healthcare systems engineering can provide answers on how the physician's office can be designed to facilitate the communication between the physician and the patient; how the encounter between a physician and patient can be designed to maximise efficacy; the effect of new technology on nursing work processes; the best team setting in an intensive care unit or emergency department; how a survey for the patients and their families be designed; how communication during a surgical procedure can be improved; how the usability and acceptance of medical devices and health information technologies can be improved for enhanced use, quality, and safety (Fowler et al, 2011).

Healthcare systems engineering from the aspect of quality engineering can provide answers on how healthcare outcomes should be measured and controlled; how quality is defined in healthcare; what the dimensions of quality are in healthcare; how control charts should be designed in order to identify rare epidemiological events; how the efficacy of healthcare systems can be compared to identify and benchmark the best systems; how design of experiment techniques can be used to develop effective clinical trials (Fowler et al, 2011).

The area of healthcare informatics can provide answers on how the healthcare delivery system can take advantage of the internet; what the issues in the management of electronic medical records are; what information and knowledge can be extracted from a massive dataset; how the information flow between healthcare providers can be designed to assure effective and timely distribution; what informatics solutions should be implemented to support healthcare delivery processes (Fowler et al, 2011).

Medical decision-making can provide answers on what the optimal timing of treatment for patients with a chronic disease such as heart disease, cancer, or diabetes is; when the optimal time to discharge a patient from a hospital in order to guarantee safety and reduce cost is; what the optimal design of an intensity-modulated radiation therapy programme is; what the best policies for organ allocation within a geographic region are; how the characteristics and preference of the patients affect their medical decisions; what the best way to use tests with imperfect sensitivity and specificity to detect and treat disease is; how treatments be used in combination to achieve a common goal such as maximising quality-adjusted life span; how limited treatment and screening resources be allocated to achieve maximum benefit to population should be allocated (Fowler et al, 2011).

Enablement of working with people stakeholders to derive realistic systems models; improvements to patient information, taking a system-wide view of patient flow and resource needs; creating virtual design alternatives to explore process options; and evaluating new process risks utilising simulation models, are some of the key critical success factors for application of a systems engineering model in healthcare and medicine (Royal Academy of Engineering, 2017).

The challenge is that while there are systems methods and tools that have the potential to make an impact in healthcare, such techniques are still not widely used in healthcare even in developed countries such as the United States of America (President's Council of Advisors on Science and Technology (PCAST), 2014).

3.2.1.2 Patient safety and security

IMPROVING PATIENT SAFETY and healthcare delivery. "It is asserted that improving integration within the intensive care unit (ICU) will lead to the desired goal of safe and effective healthcare delivery as other fields and industries have realised performance improvements by capitalising on improved information awareness, timeliness, completeness, and accuracy – attributes that are notably lacking in healthcare.

A new paradigm is needed for the design and integration of technology within the ICU to achieve the advantages of interoperability. This new paradigm is needed because today's medical systems are effectively closed proprietary systems that severely curtail the ability to extract data and information. A lesson learned is that the needs of the patient and family are not limited to improved communication but also extend beyond what people commonly consider technology-related topics.

The proposed ICU should have the environmental factors desired by patients and family members as expressed by them in the study suggesting a need for improvements in the ICU environment. They called for quieter settings and a desire for fresh air and natural light in the ICU. It is emphasised that the patient and family must be kept at the centre of the systems approach. There are no technical barriers to enabling that capability, and the payoff in terms of patient and family experience may be substantial" (Ravitz et al, 2013).

3.2.1.3 Economic and financial aspects

WHILE ADVANCES IN HEALTHCARE systems engineering can greatly increase the effectiveness and efficiency of healthcare delivery, implementing healthcare systems engineering can be costly. There is an opportunity, though, because globalisation is making way for joint ventures and foreign direct investments.

———●———

3.2.1.4 Organisational aspects

HEALTHCARE SYSTEMS engineering from the aspect of quality engineering can provide answers on how healthcare outcomes should be measured and controlled; how quality is defined in healthcare; what the dimensions of quality are in healthcare; how control charts should be designed in order to identify rare epidemiological events; how the efficacy of healthcare systems can be compared to identify and benchmark the best systems; how design of experiment techniques can be used to develop effective clinical trials (Fowler et al, 2011).

The area of healthcare informatics can provide answers on how the healthcare delivery system can take advantage of the internet; what the issues in the management of electronic medical records are; what information and knowledge can be extracted from a massive dataset; how the information flow between healthcare providers can be designed to assure effective and timely distribution; what informatics solutions should be implemented to support healthcare delivery processes (Fowler et al, 2011).

Accelerating improvements for better healthcare and lower costs through systems engineering. "Potential impact of systems engineering on different segments of the health system can be viewed in the context of systems methods and tools to address selected challenges pertaining to health systems stakeholders such as patients, small clinical practices, large healthcare organisations, and communities.

For patients as health system stakeholders, operations management can ensure that resources are available when needed; checklists or dashboards can ensure reliable care delivery; reengineering processes can incorporate patient input.

For small clinical practices as health system stakeholders, lean techniques can be employed for eliminating waste in workflows and clinical processes; human factors engineering techniques can ensure health information tools are easily usable.

For large healthcare organisations as health system stakeholders, standardised protocols that incorporate new evidence can be tailored to individual patients; predictive analytics can identify potential risks before problems occur; supply chain management can help minimise waste in supplies and pharmaceuticals. For communities as health system stakeholders, it can be modelled how policies can build on communities; operations research can identify at-risk community members and effectively deliver preventive health services; big data methods can be applied for identifying patients who need more intensive coordination of their healthcare (President's Council of Advisors on Science and Technology (PCAST), 2014).

The challenge is that while there are systems methods and tools that have the potential to make an impact in healthcare, such techniques are still not widely used in healthcare in the United States of America (President's Council of Advisors on Science and Technology (PCAST), 2014).

On healthcare reform. "Evidence shows that approximately 85 per cent of process variability can be attributed to the system and the remaining 15 per cent is attributed to random variation, and that according to the Pareto Principle only a few causes have major effects on total variation. The proposed approach as a solution to the high systemic costs of the healthcare system in the United States of America consists of three parts.

Firstly, introducing national level standards and incentives for the creation of an integrated healthcare information system will address variability from geographic and individual variability of actions by healthcare insurers, geographic variability of tort laws, and geographic and individual variability of healthcare treatment processes and levels of treatment.

Secondly, standardising external operating conditions such as passing medical malpractice liability bill using the model as the observed best practice and also passing a comprehensive national tort reform to provide a standardised framework of liability for businesses including pharmaceutical and medical technology companies will address variability from geographic variability of tort laws.

Thirdly, introducing competition for the current form of health insurance by using a novel approach in the form of a virtual Health Coverage Transaction Facilitator – Enterprise Resource Planning solution to address variability from geographic and individual variability of actions by healthcare insurers, geographic variability of tort laws, and geographic and individual variability of healthcare treatment processes and levels of treatment" (Waissi, 2010).

A systems approach to health and care design and continuous improvement. "A successful systems engineering delivery process in healthcare should focus on defining stakeholder needs and required functionality early in the development cycle, documenting requirements, then proceeding with design synthesis and system validation while considering the complete problem. Some of the critical success factors for application of a systems engineering model in healthcare include: working with people stakeholders to derive realistic systems models; improvements to patient information, clinician knowledge and impact of regulatory policy; taking a system-wide view of patient flow and resource needs; creating virtual design alternatives to explore process options; evaluating new process risks utilising simulation models" (Royal Academy of Engineering, 2017).

3.2.1.5 Socio-cultural and socio-technical aspects

FROM A CULTURAL AND societal angle, it is an advantage that there is generally increasing attention in healthcare. It is a challenge that healthcare systems engineering is not understood by many healthcare professionals in both low- and middle-income countries (LMICs) and high-income countries, and, perhaps, more so, in LMICs, as this technology cuts across the healthcare ecosystem. There is need for education and more transparency so that both the healthcare providers and consumers can be on-board to ensure buy-in, ownership, accountability and sustainability of healthcare system engineering.

Application of engineering systems models in healthcare and medicine enables improvement and impact of regulatory policies (Royal Academy of Engineering, 2017).

Healthcare public policy can provide answers on how limited resources should be allocated to control infectious diseases; how emergency items should be pre-positioned to provide effective response to disasters; whether the benefits of certain preventive treatment methods justify their costs; what the likely results from a needle exchange programme are; when schools should be closed during a pandemic influenza outbreak (Fowler et al, 2011).

In terms of socio-technical systems analysis, healthcare systems engineering can provide answers on how the physician's office can be designed to facilitate the communication between the physician and the patient; how the encounter between a physician and patient can be designed to maximise efficacy; the effect of new technology on nursing work processes; the best team setting in an intensive care unit or emergency department; how a survey for the patients and their families be designed; how communication during a surgical procedure can be improved; how the usability and acceptance of medical devices and health information technologies can be improved for enhanced use, quality, and safety (Fowler et al, 2011).

———◉———

3.2.1.6 Legal and regulatory aspects

HEALTHCARE PUBLIC POLICY can provide answers on how limited resources should be allocated to control infectious diseases; how emergency items should be pre-positioned to provide effective response to disasters; whether the benefits of certain preventive treatment methods justify their costs; what the likely results from a needle exchange programme are; when schools should be closed during a pandemic influenza outbreak" (Fowler et al, 2011).

———◉———

3.2.2 Conclusion

IT IS ASSERTED THAT improving integration within the ICU will lead to the desired goal of safe and effective healthcare delivery as other fields and industries have realised performance improvements by capitalising on improved information awareness, timeliness, completeness, and accuracy – attributes that are notably lacking in healthcare. A new paradigm is needed for the design and integration of technology within the ICU to achieve the advantages of interoperability. This new paradigm is needed because today's medical systems are effectively closed proprietary systems that severely curtail the ability to extract data and information. A lesson learned is that the needs of the patient and family are not limited to improved communication but also extend beyond what people commonly consider technology-related topics. The proposed ICU should have the environmental factors desired by patients and family members as expressed by them in the study suggesting a need for improvements in the ICU environment. They called for quieter settings and a desire for fresh air and natural light in the ICU. It is emphasised that the patient and family must be kept at the centre of the systems approach. There are no technical barriers to enabling that capability and the payoff in terms of patient and family experience may be substantial (Ravitz et al, 2013).

A successful systems engineering delivery process in healthcare should focus on defining stakeholder needs and required functionality early in the development cycle, documenting requirements, then proceeding with design synthesis and system validation while considering the complete problem (Royal Academy of Engineering, 2017).

REFERENCES

Al-Fadel, H.O. (2004) *Clinical engineering in the Middle East*. In: Dyro, Iadanza & Dyro; Clinical Engineering Handbook, pp. 97-98. Academic Press. https://doi.org/10.1016/B978-012226570-9/50032-6

Fernandez, F. & Pallis, G.C. (2014) *Opportunity and challenges of the Internet of things for healthcare: systems engineering perspective*. IEEE 4th International Conference on Wireless Mobile Communication and Healthcare – Transforming Healthcare Through Innovations in Mobile and Wireless Technologies (MOBIHEALTH).

Fowler, J.W. et al. (2011) An introduction to a new journal for healthcare systems engineering. *IIE Transactions on Healthcare Systems Engineering*, 1, 1-5.

Gentles, B. (2004) *Clinical engineering in Canada*. In: Dyro, Iadanza & Dyro; Clinical Engineering Handbook, pp. 62-64.

Girling, W. (2020) *Clinical engineering is reshaping digital healthcare*. Healthcare

Grimes, S. (2004) The future of clinical engineering: the challenge of change. *IEEE Engineering in Medicine and Biology Magazine*, 22(2), 91-99.

Mayo Clinic (2021) *Science of health care delivery*. May Foundation for Medical Education and Research (MFMER).

McCulloch, G.M. & Tegethoff, G. (2013) Meaningful use and its impact on healthcare technology management. *Biomedical Instrumentation & Technology*. Doi: 10.2345/0899-8205-47.1.30

Murray, M. & Berwick, D.M. (2003) Advanced access: reducing waiting and delays in primary care. *Journal of the American Medical Association*, 289(8), 1035-1040.

Nunziata, E. & Sumalgy, M. (2004) *Clinical engineering in Mozambique*. In: Dyro, Iadanza & Dyro; Clinical Engineering Handbook, pp. 93-97.

President's Council of Advisors on Science and Technology (PCAST) (2014) *Report to the president - better health care and lower costs: accelerating improvement through systems engineering.* Executive Office of the President of the United States.

Raitz, A.D. et al. (2013) Systems approach and systems engineering applied to health care: improving patient safety and health care delivery. Johns Hopkins APL Technical Digest, 31 (4), 354-365.

Reid, P.P., et al. (2005) Building a better delivery system: a new engineering/health care partnership. National Academy of Engineering and Institute of Medicine of the National Academies.

Royal Academy of Engineering (2017) *Engineering better care: a systems approach to health and care design and continuous improvement.* London

Waissi, G. (2010) *On healthcare reform – a systems engineering approach.* Decision Sciences Institute (DSI) Conference Proceedings, San Diego.

Don't miss out!

Visit the website below and you can sign up to receive emails whenever Mbuso Mabuza publishes a new book. There's no charge and no obligation.

https://books2read.com/r/B-A-JPJL-IHSIC

BOOKS 2 READ

Connecting independent readers to independent writers.

Did you love *Health Systems Engineering: Building A Better Healthcare Delivery System*? Then you should read *Ethics, Qualitative And Quantitative Methods In Public Health Research*[1] by Mbuso Mabuza!

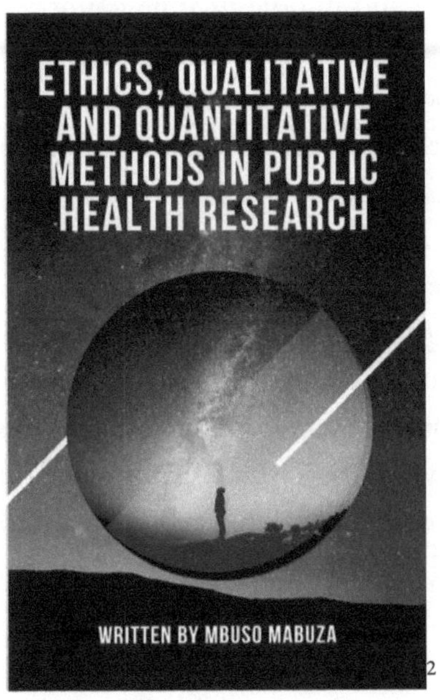

[2]

This book provides an introduction to ethics, research design as the most important part of the qualitative research process, the importance of theoretical frameworks and the relationship between the researcher and the researched in the qualitative research process.

It also provides an introduction to epidemiological research and statistical methods covering key concepts and all the main types of epidemiological study. It elicits a critical understanding of the purpose and context of quantitative research including the basis for selecting appropriate research designs from a thorough grounding in the uses and methods of epidemiology; key statistical concepts and techniques

1. https://books2read.com/u/mY8RRx

2. https://books2read.com/u/mY8RRx

needed for the basic analysis of data; critical evaluation of statistical and epidemiological techniques in health research.

The book has been designed around a number of core published information dealing with various topics from the United Kingdom, Europe and the low- and middle-income countries. These studies have been chosen to introduce you to a wide range of study methods. The main intriguing aspects of their design provide examples which are used to help you understand the fundamental principles of good research, and to practise these techniques yourself.

The book is divided into two sections. Section 1 focuses on ethics and qualitative methods in public health research. This section is organised according to the following chapters: ethics and introduction to qualitative research; qualitative research study design; qualitative methods – participant observation; qualitative methods – interviews, texts, and qualitative diaries; participatory and action research; data analysis – coding, storing and managing qualitative data; analysis – interpretation; validity and presentation of findings to different audiences.

Section 2 of this book focuses on quantitative methods in public health research. This section is divided into the following chapters: scientific method and introductory concepts; routine data sources and descriptive epidemiology; surveys; cohort studies; case-control studies; and critical appraisal of research evidence.

This book will be an invaluable resource for health professionals, researchers, statisticians, data scientists, health programmers, policymakers, medical students, graduate and postgraduate students in public health and related disciplines.

Also by Mbuso Mabuza

A Healthy Mind And Best You: Achieving Great Results in Every Aspect of Your Life

Purposeful And Better You

Sustainable Development Calls for Effective Strategic Leadership for Efficient Health Systems

Health Promotion In Low Socioeconomic Settings

Medicine and Sociology of Health

Qualitative Methods In Public Health Research

Global Health Disaster Management

Global Health Policy And Programme Challenges

The Journey of Life Has a Gift of Purpose

Epidemiological Research

Ethics, Qualitative And Quantitative Methods In Public Health Research

When Love Lasts

Blockchain Technology In Healthcare

Virtual and Augmented Reality in Healthcare

Data Analytics and Healthcare Informatics

How To Improve The Way You Think

Health Systems Engineering: Building A Better Healthcare Delivery System

Artificial Intelligence In Drug Discovery And Development

About the Author

Dr Mbuso Mabuza is a highly motivated life-long learner and multi-skilled global health professional. Dr Mabuza's mission is to improve health outcomes and to expand quality healthcare experiences amongst all groups of people and influence change and innovation.